Penguin Books

Physical Fitness: XBX

# The
# Royal Canadian Air Force

# XBX Plan
# for Physical Fitness
# for Women

Penguin Books

PENGUIN BOOKS

Published by the Penguin Group
Penguin Books Ltd, 27 Wrights Lane, London W8 5TZ, England
Penguin Books USA Inc., 375 Hudson Street, New York, New York 10014, USA
Penguin Books Australia Ltd, Ringwood, Victoria, Australia
Penguin Books Canada Ltd, 10 Alcorn Avenue, Toronto, Ontario, Canada M4V 3B2
Penguin Books (NZ) Ltd, 182–190 Wairau Road, Auckland 10, New Zealand

Penguin Books Ltd, Registered Offices: Harmondsworth, Middlesex, England

5BX first published by the R.C.A.F. 1958
XBX first published by the R.C.A.F. 1960
Published in one volume in Penguin Books 1964
This separate volume published 1986
10 9 8 7 6

Photographs by Colin Thomas
Crown Copyright © Queen's Printer, Canada, 1958, 1960
Reproduced by permission
All rights reserved

Printed in England by Clays Ltd, St Ives plc
Set in Linotron Ehrhardt

# Contents

# Foreword

This is an age in which, even in the country, more and more people go everywhere on wheels. Keeping fit has become a universal problem. Though they may not be willing to spend time and money at a gymnasium and have no ambitions in the sphere of the 'body beautiful', very many people are nevertheless worried today about their figures and their general state of health.

The system of exercises detailed in this book presents an exceedingly simple answer to the problem. These plans were developed by the Royal Canadian Air Force in order to keep personnel at a peak of physical fitness, ready to face sudden demands for energy after long periods of inactivity. When they were made available to the general public, the two booklets of exercises rapidly became bestsellers all over North America. Their publication in Penguins will enable them to reach an even wider audience.

These exercises are specially designed for those who are pressed for time, whose work is mainly sedentary, and who have neither the space nor the taste for formal games or walks; for city-dwellers (in particular) who, even if they hardly ever go to the shops without a car, may occasionally have to sprint for a bus or climb stairs when the lift is out of order; and for those who are becoming aware of 'middle-aged spread' or of the strain of work, but are disinclined to take very strong action.

The XBX plan, as these exercises are called, is graded progressively and the performer is not expected to go beyond the simpler movements at the beginning of the course until he or she can do them without difficulty in the time set. The pace of progress and the degree of fitness are entirely up to the performer. In this way it has been proved that adequate fitness can be achieved by easy stages, in very little space and without exaggerated exertion, at the cost of only a few minutes each day. Above all this system does not reach too high. It aims to provide the right degree of fitness for all normal purposes, without arousing any anxiety about Olympic standards of training.

The XBX is ideal for anyone who simply wants to get fit, look fit, feel fit, and stay fit.

# Acknowledgements

The R.C.A.F. acknowledges the contribution made to the preparation of the XBX Pamphlet by N. J. Ashton, B.Sc., M.S., Physical Education Specialist.

# Introduction

## Why You Should Be Fit

Research has shown that the physically fit person is able to withstand fatigue for longer periods than the unfit; that the physically fit person is better equipped to tolerate physical stress; that the physically fit person has a stronger and more efficient heart; and that there is a relationship between good mental alertness, absence of nervous tension, and physical fitness.

Remember that:

(1) weak stomach muscles cause sagging abdomens; and
(2) weak back muscles are a major cause of back pain.

There are countless reasons for being fit. *You* know how you feel. *Everyone* knows how you look. Regular exercise can improve your sense of well-being and your appearance. Fitness is necessary for the fullest enjoyment of living.

## Weight Control

The major purpose of weight control is to reduce the amount of fat on the body and to increase the amount of muscle. It is, in reality, a programme of fat control rather than weight control. This control can be exerted only by coupling a sensible dietary programme with a regular, balanced programme of exercise.

When we eat, the food is used, stored, or discarded. The body stores fuel, or calories, as fat. The more fuel we consume, and the less of it we use, then the more of it that is stored in the body in the form of fat. The human body is not like a car's petrol tank that will overflow when full. Our bodies accept all the calories that we put into them, and store those which we do not use.

For example, if you eat food that has a value of 3,000 calories and use only 2,600 of them in your activity, then the remaining 400 calories are stored in the body. Every time you accumulate about 4,000 of these calories you will notice an extra pound of weight on the scales.

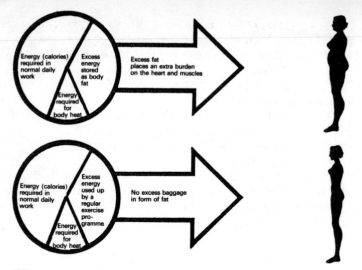

When you exercise you burn calories. Energy used in this way will result in muscle development. As muscle is slightly heavier than fat, you may very well notice an increase in your weight rather than a reduction. However it must be stressed that this muscle weight is useful weight and will improve the way you look and feel.

Research has shown clearly that the most effective way of taking off weight and keeping it off is through a programme which combines exercise and diet.

## Live To Be Fit and Be Fit To Live

This book is concerned primarily with the habits of exercise and diet as steps on the road to fitness. Many more ways and means exist which can become habits that will also contribute to this goal. Try to make some of these a part of your daily living and you will soon find that without conscious effort, or extra 'work', you are gaining many benefits.

Walking is an excellent exercise if done at a faster pace than a slow shuffle. If you use public transport, do not use the nearest or most convenient stop, but get on or off a few streets away and walk briskly. Walk to the corner shop or post box rather than use your car. At every opportunity, walk rather than ride. Climb a few flights of stairs instead of using the lift or escalator.

Use your muscles for lifting objects when you are able, rather than pushing them. Even an everyday practice like drying yourself with a towel after bathing can become a fitness activity. Rub down briskly rather than dabbing.

While sitting at a desk or table you can aid posture and tone up muscles. Sit tall with your back straight; do not slump with round back and shoulders, and head forward. To tone up the shoulder girdle and arm muscles: sit erect, place hands on desk, palms down, elbows bent, and press down, trying to lift body from chair. Hold the pressure for a few seconds. Repeat two or three times a day.

When standing, sitting, or lying, tense the muscles of the abdomen and hold for about six seconds. Do this a few times each day. Constantly think of how you look, and walk tall and sit tall, always attempting to maintain a good postural position.

## Rest, Relaxation, and Revitalization

It is just as important that your body receives adequate rest as it is that it be exercised. Sleep requirements vary from person to person and each person is his own best judge of these needs. The important thing is to awake refreshed and revitalized. A few tips on getting the most from your bedtime hours:

(1) keep the room as dark as possible;
(2) do not take your problems to bed with you – if you must think, think calm, restful thoughts;
(3) mild exercise before retiring may be helpful;
(4) if you are hungry, have a light snack or a warm, non-stimulating beverage.

Relaxation, both mental and physical, is becoming more and more essential in the fast moving, hurly-burly world in which we live. Many emotional tensions are reflected in physical tensions, both organic and muscular.

You can consciously reduce both forms of tension. Physically you can learn to relax muscle groups. A simple illustration is this: hold your hands in front of you, tighten up the muscles of the forearms so that the hands and fingers are straight, abruptly relax them so that the hands fall limply. Try this with other muscles – tighten – then relax. Stretch, writhe, and wriggle yourself into a relaxed state.

For mental relaxation try consciously to think pleasant and restful thoughts, ignoring for a while the troubles of the day. Healthy forms of recreation (picnics, golf, etc.) are fine ways to release not only the physical tensions, but some of the mental ones as well.

## Exercise and the Heart

There are many misconceptions about exercise and its effect upon the heart. 'Exercise is harmful.' Nonsense. There is no evidence to support this contention. There is a large body of opinion which holds that exercise, appropriate to age and physical condition, continued through your life span, will help to reduce the possibility of heart and blood vessel disease. Exercise, in mild form of course, is recommended as part of the recuperative phase in cases of heart or coronary disease. Evidence is also on hand that indicates exercise is beneficial to the function of the cardio-vascular system.

A healthy heart can obtain many benefits from a good conditioning programme. Research has shown that the heart of a trained person has a smaller acceleration of pulse rate under stress, and that it returns more rapidly to its normal rate afterwards than that of an untrained person; that it pumps more blood per beat at rest, and that it can pump more during exercise; that it has more richly developed small blood vessels supplying the heart muscle and that it functions more efficiently. An efficient cardio-vascular system means a better supply of food and oxygen to the muscles (as blood is the carrier of these items) and a quicker recuperation after exertion, be it work, play, or exercise.

**A cautionary note:** persons over thirty-five years of age, and anyone who suspects that they may have something wrong with their heart, should have a thorough medical examination before engaging in a vigorous exercise programme. Experts have noted that a heart already injured by disease will suffer extra abuse through extreme forms of exercise. Sudden violent exertion after a period of inactivity is to be avoided.

## Exercise, Strength, and Endurance

The strength and endurance of the body can be increased through regular exercise. Such improvements are primarily localized in the muscles and organs which are exercised – one cannot strengthen the arms and shoulders by exercising the legs. To improve the condition of all muscles one must undertake a programme which will provide them all with work.

The strength of a muscle is measured by the amount of force that that muscle can exert and is dependent upon the size and number of muscle fibres that can be brought into action at any one time and the frequency of the nerve impulses to them.

Endurance is concerned with the ability to repeat an action over and over again, or to sustain a muscular contraction.

Since the fuel for muscular contraction is carried in the blood, endurance is chiefly dependent upon the functioning of the cardio-respiratory system (heart, blood vessels, and lungs) – that is, the ability of the body to transport food and oxygen to the muscles, and waste products away from them, efficiently.

The human body requires proper use to function efficiently and endure. The body is very different from a machine that wears out with use. Most persons have noted how the muscles of an arm or a leg in a cast become smaller and weaker the longer the arm or leg remains so encased. While this is a dramatic example it is in effect what happens to the muscles of the body in a milder way when these muscles are not used enough. Exercise over and above the normal demands of daily living is essential to the development of an efficient, strong, and durable body. The resultant more pleasing appearance and sense of well-being are added benefits that cannot be over-looked.

## Caution – before you start

If you have any doubt as to your capability to undertake this programme, *see your medical adviser*. You should not perform fast, vigorous, or highly competitive physical activity without gradually developing, and continuously maintaining, an adequate level of physical fitness, particularly if you are over the age of 30.

# The XBX Plan for Women

## Your Appearance

Your appearance is controlled by the bony frame of your body, and by the proportions of fat and muscle which you have added to it. You cannot do anything about your skeleton, but you can, and should, do something about the fat and muscle.

All of us require a certain amount of fat on and in our bodies for functional reasons. Fat softens the bony contours of the body; it helps to keep the body temperature constant; and it acts as an energy storage vault. Fat appears in layers on the outside of the body, covers and lines the internal organs – the heart and blood vessels, for example – and it also makes up a part of muscle.

Except for certain neurotic or glandular conditions, people are over-fat because they over-eat and under-exercise.

Muscle is the other controllable factor in the appearance. When we are young we are fairly active; the muscles of our bodies are used and they retain that pleasing firmness – muscle tone. The less we exercise muscles the softer and more flabby they become. They become small with disuse, less elastic, and much weaker. Much of what is considered fatness in the abdominal region is nothing more than weak stomach muscles which permit the internal organs to sag forward. Your muscles perform the same function as a girdle – keep them as resilient as your foundation garment.

Because the condition of your muscles is so important to the way you look and feel, diet alone is not the best method for trying to improve your body measurements. The best method is a combination of diet and exercise. A thigh that is made up of little muscle and a lot of fat may have the same measurement as one that has firm muscle and a light fat layer, but – let's face it – it is just not the same thigh.

Do not confuse good muscle tone with bulky, unsightly muscles. The XBX is designed to firm your muscles – not to convert you into a muscled woman.

## Diet

For many women, the knowledge that they have gained a few pounds, or added a few inches, causes what may be called the 'diet reflex'. Without pause to consult a medical expert they resort immediately to their favourite diet, which is more usually a fast. If you wish to go on a stringent diet – consult your doctor first.

As a rule you can avoid the need to resort to a strict reduction of food intake by the constant use of sensible dietary habits. In the normal individual, fat is added to the body very slowly. It may be several weeks or even months before you notice this gradual accumulation. You cannot hope to take this fat off and keep it off without making subtle changes in eating and exercise habits. After a 'crash diet', you will undoubtedly return to your old habits and in a few weeks you will note that *it* is back again once more.

A slight change in diet (along with XBX) can take off, and keep off, several pounds of excess fat over a period of time. For example, if you eat bread with your meals, eat one slice less; add a little less sugar, or none at all, to your tea or coffee. The calories so avoided each day add up to several thousand in a few months and may be the difference between the way you look and feel and the way you would like to look and feel. By the time you have arrived at the condition you desire your habits will have been changed enough so that you will probably not slip back into the old ones.

## What You Can Do About Fitness

Unless you are engaged in a full-time programme of conditioning for athletic endeavours you should take part in some form of active exercise.

The average woman is engaged in one of three activities daily – school, employment, or housework. None of these provides the balanced activity for the body that is desirable for good physical fitness. Housework, for example, though it may involve a good deal of hard physical labour, does not take into account the flexibility of the muscles, nor does it work all the muscles of the body. Day after day you do the same things. The muscles that work get plenty of exercise; the others get little or none.

The same facts that are true of housework also hold true for most sports. Sports make specific contributions to fitness but do not condition the whole body. Most people taking part in a recreational sport do not pursue it vigorously enough to develop adequate levels of fitness. Before they become completely effective, even those sports which can produce all-round fitness require more skill than the average person possesses and more time than the average person can devote to them.

No matter what you do in your daily life you probably need a good, balanced programme of exercise which will enable you to become the person you want to be.

## Why XBX Was Developed

Research has indicated that everyone – male and female, young and old – is in need of some form of regular, vigorous, physical activity. As more and more labour-saving devices are put into general use, as more and more people watch more and more television, films, and sports events, the amount of physical effort expended by the average person decreases continually.

An analysis of the exercise needs of Canadians was conducted by R.C.A.F. specialists and led to the development of the 5BX programme for men. XBX is the complementary programme for women.

The R.C.A.F. analysis indicated three major deterrents to regular exercise:

(1) a great majority of people would like to exercise, but do not know how to go about it – what to do, how to do it, how often, how to progress, or how far to progress;

(2) most exercise programmes call for the use of equipment and gymnasiums which are not always available; and

(3) most exercise programmes call for a great expenditure of time, which most people cannot spare.

Clearly a programme which resolves these problems is required.

The XBX tells you what to do, where to start, how fast you progress, and how far you should progress to achieve a desirable level of physical fitness. It requires no equipment and very little space, and takes only twelve minutes a day.

## How XBX Was Developed

XBX is the product of extensive research into the problems of physical fitness for girls and women, the research having been conducted at several R.C.A.F. stations and in the later stages having included sections of the civilian population. Over 600 girls and women of all ages participated in the project and the R.C.A.F. is indebted to them for their contributions to the programme.

The first step in the project was the administration of a series of physical fitness tests. The tests included an examination of muscular strength and endurance, testing of heart response to activity, and measurement of fat layers. From the results of these tests the physical fitness needs of women were analysed. Experiments were carried out with a wide variety of exercises to determine those most effective in producing the desired results. Many of these exercises were discarded as ineffectual. The ten exercises of XBX provided the most balanced and effective programme.

The time limits for each exercise were varied until the optimum time for good results was determined, and the tests were conducted to arrive at the number of times each exercise could be done, and should be done, within the time limits.

Several hundred women used the first experimental exercise programmes and periodic tests showed that XBX was an effective plan to improve levels of general fitness.

The programme was then distributed to groups and to individuals across Canada for further trial and comment. Further modifications in the plan were made on the basis of this final field trial. The results of this research are presented in this book – the R.C.A.F. XBX Plan for Physical Fitness.

**What the XBX Plan Is**

The XBX Plan is a physical fitness programme composed of four charts of ten exercises, arranged in progressive order of difficulty. The ten exercises on each chart are always performed in the same order, and in the same maximum time limits.

The charts are divided into levels. There are 48 levels in all, 12 in each chart. The levels are numbered consecutively, starting with 1 at the bottom of Chart One and ending with 48 at the top of Chart Four.

In addition to the regular exercises, two supplementary exercises are available for Charts One, Two, and Three. These exercises are for the muscles of the feet and ankles and for those muscles which assist in the maintenance of good posture.

## How XBX Works

Any exercise plan or programme should work on the basis of an easy start and gradual progression. As physical fitness improves, the work load is increased. The XBX approach to exercise follows these principles. XBX incorporates two methods to make the work load greater:

(1) the time limit for each exercise remains the same in all charts, but the number of times the exercise is performed within this time limit is increased at each level within each chart; and

(2) the exercises are made more difficult from each chart to the next higher one.

On each chart you do the same exercises at each of the twelve levels but increase the number of times you do them. As you move to the next higher chart the exercises are basically the same but have been modified and made slightly more demanding.

The XBX has been planned for gradual, painless progression. Follow the plan as outlined in the booklet; do not skip levels; do not progress faster than is recommended.

## What the Exercises Are For

The XBX will improve your general physical condition by (1) increasing muscle tone; (2) increasing muscular strength; (3) increasing muscular endurance; (4) increasing flexibility; and (5) increasing the efficiency of your heart. Each exercise is included because of its contribution in one or more of these areas.

**The first four exercises** are primarily to improve and maintain flexibility and mobility in those areas of the body which are usually neglected. They also serve as a warm-up for the more strenuous exercises which follow.

**Exercise Five** is for strengthening the abdominal region and the muscles of the fronts of the thighs.

**Exercise Six** exercises the long muscles of the back, the buttocks, and the backs of the thighs.

**Exercise Seven** concentrates on the muscles on the sides of the thighs. These muscles get very little work in routine daily activities, or indeed in most sports.

# Chart 2

| Level | 1 | 2 | 3 | 4 | 5 | 6 | 7 | 8 | 9 | 10 | 8a | 8b |
|---|---|---|---|---|---|---|---|---|---|---|---|---|
| | **Exercise** | | | | | | | | | | | |
| **24** | 15 | 16 | 12 | 30 | 35 | 38 | 50 | 28 | 20 | 210 | 40 | 36 |
| **23** | 15 | 16 | 12 | 30 | 33 | 36 | 48 | 26 | 18 | 200 | 38 | 34 |
| **22** | 15 | 16 | 12 | 30 | 31 | 34 | 46 | 24 | 18 | 200 | 36 | 32 |
| **21** | 13 | 14 | 11 | 26 | 29 | 32 | 44 | 23 | 16 | 190 | 33 | 29 |
| **20** | 13 | 14 | 11 | 26 | 27 | 31 | 42 | 21 | 16 | 175 | 31 | 27 |
| **19** | 13 | 14 | 11 | 26 | 24 | 29 | 40 | 20 | 14 | 160 | 28 | 24 |
| **18** | 12 | 12 | 9 | 20 | 22 | 27 | 38 | 18 | 14 | 150 | 25 | 22 |
| **17** | 12 | 12 | 9 | 20 | 19 | 24 | 36 | 16 | 12 | 150 | 22 | 20 |
| **16** | 12 | 12 | 9 | 20 | 16 | 21 | 34 | 14 | 10 | 140 | 19 | 19 |
| **15** | 10 | 10 | 7 | 18 | 14 | 18 | 32 | 12 | 10 | 130 | 17 | 15 |
| **14** | 10 | 10 | 7 | 18 | 11 | 15 | 30 | 10 | 8 | 120 | 14 | 13 |
| **13** | 10 | 10 | 7 | 18 | 9 | 12 | 28 | 8 | 8 | 120 | 12 | 12 |
| Minutes for each exercise | 2 | | | | 2 | 1 | 1 | 2 | 1 | 3 | 1 | 1 |

Recommended number of days at each level [    ]

**Exercise Eight** is primarily for the arms, shoulders, and chest, but at the same time exercises the back and abdomen.

**Exercise Nine** is partly for flexibility in the waist area and for strengthening the muscles of the hips and sides.

**Exercise Ten**, the stationary run with jumping, while exercising the legs, is primarily for the conditioning of the heart and lungs.

**The two supplementary exercises** are included for those who wish to do a little more. One exercise is for strengthening the muscles of the feet and the ankle joint. The other is for those muscles of the back and abdomen which assist in the maintenance of posture.

## What the Charts Mean

Below is an explanation of what the chart pages mean. Check the paragraph headings with the sample chart above.

## My Progress

| Level | Started | Finished | Comments |
|---|---|---|---|
| **24** | | | |
| **23** | | | |
| **22** | | | |
| **22** | | | |
| **21** | | | |
| **20** | | | |
| **19** | | | |
| **18** | | | |
| **17** | | | |
| **16** | | | |
| **15** | | | |
| **14** | | | |
| **13** | | | |

| | Date | Height | Weight | Waist | Hips | Bust |
|---|---|---|---|---|---|---|
| My aim | | | | | | |
| Start | | | | | | |
| Finish | | | | | | |

**Exercise**  The numbers across the tops of the charts are the exercise numbers from 1 to 10. The column headed 1 refers to Exercise One, and so on. The exercises are described and illustrated in the four or five pages following each chart. Exercises 8A and 8B are the supplementary exercises described on pages 89–95. If you choose to do these, do them between Exercises Eight and Nine.

**Level**  The numbers along the left side of the chart are the levels of the programme, and each refers to the line of numbers beside it under the exercise headings. For example at Level 14 you do Exercise Three seven times, Exercise Six fifteen times, and so on.

**Minutes for Each Exercise**  The allotted time for each exercise is shown here. The exercises numbered 1 to 4 are the warm-up and all four are to be completed within two minutes, or about a half minute each. Other examples: Exercise Five takes two minutes and

Exercise Six takes one minute. The total time for each level of ten exercises is twelve minutes. It is important that all the exercises be done within this total time limit. Do not move up to the next level until you can do your present level, without excessive strain or fatigue, in the twelve minutes.

**Recommended Number of Days at Each Level**  Record in the box provided on each chart page the number of days it is recommended that you spend at each level before progressing to the next. (See instructions for using the plan on page 24.)

**My Progress**  This chart is provided to enable you to keep an accurate record of your progress on the way to your physical fitness goal. Record the dates you started and finished each level. Make a note of how you felt as you did the exercises. To use the bottom chart, select a reasonable aim for yourself in terms of body measurements and record this in the boxes marked 'My aim'. Then record your present measurements on the Start line. When you have completed the exercise chart, note your latest measurements on the line labelled Finish. The finish line on one chart will be the start line on the next.

*Note:* do not expect startling results. Fitness takes time and persistence. Couple your XBX programme with a good diet, and your progress will be steady.


**Your Fitness Goal**

As is explained in the instructions for the use of the programme on page 24 each age group is given a physical fitness goal to attain; that is, a level which they should try to reach.

The goals indicated in this plan are based on the average achievements of girls and women who have participated in it. Your goal, then, is the level of fitness that the average girl or woman of your age reached without undue stress, strain, or fatigue.

With every average, there are individuals who surpass it, and those who fall below it. In terms of the XBX plan and the goals, this means that there will be some women who are capable of progressing beyond the goal indicated, and on the other hand, there will be persons who will never attain this average level.

If you feel able to move further through the charts than your goal, by all means do so. If, on the contrary, you experience great difficulty in approaching this level you should stop at a level which you feel to be within your capability. It is impossible to predict accurately a level for each individual who uses this programme. Use the goals as guides, and apply them with common sense.

From time to time as you progress through the levels you may have difficulty with a particular level or exercise. If so, proceed slowly but keep working at it. (These 'plateaux' may occur anywhere in the progression.) Generally you will be able to move ahead after a few days at this level. If you cannot, then you have probably arrived at your potential physical fitness level in so far as this particular programme is concerned.

## Caution

If for any reason you stop doing XBX for more than two weeks because of illness, vacation, or any other cause – *do not* restart at the level you had attained before stopping. *Do* drop back several levels or to the next lower chart until you find a level which you can do fairly easily. Physical fitness is lost during long periods of inactivity. This is particularly true if the inactivity is caused by illness.

## Instructions for Using the XBX Plan

First select *your goal* for your age from the table opposite. Locate this level in the charts which follow. Mark it in some way – circle it or underline it.

Record the recommended minimum number of days at each level in the box provided on each chart page. For example if you are 28 years of age, your goal is Level 30 on Chart Three and you spend *at least* two days doing each level on Chart One, three days at each level on Chart Two, and five days at each level on Chart Three. Do not move faster than the recommended rate.

## To Start and Progress

Start at Level One, which is at the bottom of Chart One. When you can do this level without strain and in twelve minutes move up to Level Two. Continue through the levels and charts in this way until you reach the goal level recommended for your age group, or until you feel you are exercising at your maximum capacity.

## When You Reach Your Goal

Once you have reached your goal you should require only three exercise periods a week to maintain it.

| If your age is (years) | Your goal is Level | Recommended minimum number of days at each level on | | | |
|---|---|---|---|---|---|
| | | Chart 1 | Chart 2 | Chart 3 | Chart 4 |
| 7–8 | 30 | 1 | 1 | 2 | – |
| 9–10 | 34 | 1 | 1 | 2 | – |
| 11–12 | 38 | 1 | 1 | 2 | 3 |
| 13–14 | 41 | 1 | 1 | 2 | 3 |
| 15–17 | 44 | 1 | 1 | 2 | 3 |
| 18–19 | 40 | 1 | 2 | 3 | 4 |
| 20–25 | 35 | 1 | 2 | 3 | – |
| 26–30 | 30 | 2 | 3 | 5 | – |
| 31–5 | 26 | 2 | 4 | 6 | – |
| 36–40 | 22 | 4 | 6 | – | – |
| 41–5 | 19 | 5 | 7 | – | – |
| 46–50 | 16 | 7 | 8 | – | – |
| 51–5 | 11 | 8 | – | – | – |

# Chart 1

Handwritten column labels (left to right): TOES · KNEES · SIDE BENDS · ARMS · PARTIAL SIT-UPS · CHEST + LEG · SIDE LEG · PUSH-UPS · LEG-LIFTING · RUN + HOP

| Level | Exercise | | | | | | | | | | | |
|---|---|---|---|---|---|---|---|---|---|---|---|---|
| | 1 | 2 | 3 | 4 | 5 | 6 | 7 | 8 | 9 | 10 | 8a | 8b |
| 12 | 9 | 8 | 10 | 40 | 26 | 20 | 30 | 14 | 14 | 170 | 18 | 20 |
| 11 | 9 | 8 | 10 | 40 | 24 | 18 | 28 | 13 | 14 | 160 | 17 | 18 |
| 10 | 9 | 8 | 10 | 40 | 22 | 16 | 26 | 12 | 12 | 150 | 16 | 17 |
| 9 | 7 | 7 | 8 | 36 | 20 | 14 | 24 | 10 | 11 | 140 | 14 | 15 |
| 8 | 7 | 7 | 8 | 36 | 18 | 12 | 20 | 9 | 10 | 125 | 13 | 14 |
| 7 | 7 | 7 | 8 | 36 | 16 | 12 | 18 | 8 | 10 | 115 | 11 | 12 |
| 6 | 5 | 5 | 7 | 28 | 14 | 10 | 16 | 7 | 8 | 100 | 10 | 11 |
| 5 | 5 | 5 | 7 | 28 | 12 | 8 | 14 | 6 | 6 | 90 | 8 | 9 |
| 4 | 5 | 5 | 7 | 28 | 10 | 8 | 10 | 5 | 6 | 80 | 7 | 8 |
| 3 | 3 | 4 | 5 | 24 | 8 | 6 | 8 | 4 | 4 | 70 | 6 | 6 |
| 2 | 3 | 4 | 5 | 24 | 6 | 4 | 6 | 3 | 3 | 60 | 5 | 5 |
| 1 | 3 | 4 | 5 | 24 | 4 | 4 | 4 | 3 | 2 | 50 | 4 | 3 |
| Minutes for each exercise | | 2 | | | 2 | 1 | 1 | 2 | 1 | 3 | 1 | 1 |

Recommended number of days at each level ☐

## My Progress

| Level | Started | Finished | Comments |
|-------|---------|----------|----------|
| 12 | _____ | _____ | _____ |
| 11 | _____ | _____ | _____ |
| 10 | _____ | _____ | _____ |
| 9 | _____ | _____ | _____ |
| 8 | _____ | _____ | _____ |
| 7 | _____ | _____ | _____ |
| 6 | _____ | _____ | _____ |
| 5 | _____ | _____ | _____ |
| 4 | _____ | _____ | _____ |
| 3 | _____ | _____ | _____ |
| 2 | _____ | _____ | _____ |
| 1 | _____ | _____ | _____ |

| | Date | Height | Weight | Waist | Hips | Bust |
|--------|------|--------|--------|-------|------|------|
| My aim | _____ | _____ | _____ | _____ | _____ | _____ |
| Start | _____ | _____ | _____ | _____ | _____ | _____ |
| Finish | _____ | _____ | _____ | _____ | _____ | _____ |

## 1  Toe touching

**Start** Stand erect, feet 12 inches apart, arms over head.

Bend forward to touch floor between feet. Do not try to keep knees straight.

Return to starting position.

**Count** Each return to starting position counts one.

## 2  Knee raising

**Start** Stand erect, hands at sides, feet together.

Raise left knee as high as possible, grasping knee and shin with hands. Pull leg towards body. Keep back straight throughout. Lower foot to floor.

Repeat with right leg. Continue by alternating legs – left then right.

**Count** Left and right knee raises count one.

CHART I

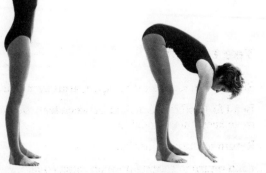

1

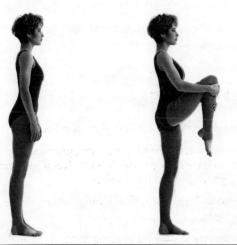

2

## 3  Lateral bending

**Start**  Stand erect, feet 12 inches apart, hands at sides.

Keeping back straight, bend sidewards from waist to left.
Slide left hand down leg as far as possible.

Return to starting position and bend to right side.
Continue by alternating to left then right.

**Count**  Bends to the left and right count one.

CHART I

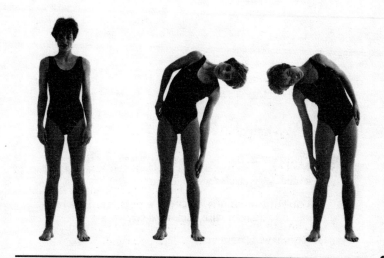

3

## 4  Arm circling

Stand erect, feet 12 inches apart, arms at sides.

Make large circles with left arm.

Do one quarter of total count with forward circles and one quarter with backward circles.

Repeat with right arm.

**Count** A full arm circle counts one.

CHART I

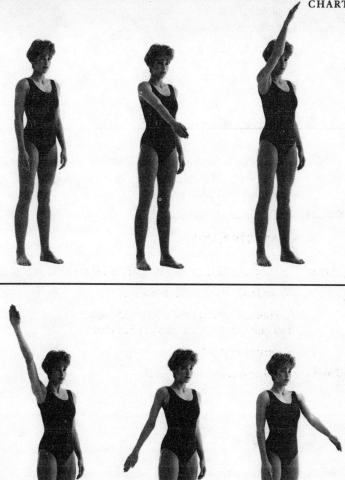

4

## 5  Partial sit-ups

**Start**  Lie on back, legs straight and together, arms at sides.

Raise head and shoulders from floor until you can see your heels. Lower head to floor.

**Count**  Each partial sit-up counts one.

## 6  Chest and leg raising

**Start**  Lie face down, arms along sides, hands under thighs, palms pressing against thighs.

Raise head, shoulders, and left leg as high as possible from floor. Keep leg straight. Lower to floor.

Repeat raising head, shoulders, and right leg. Continue by alternating legs, left then right.

**Count**  Each chest and leg raise counts one.

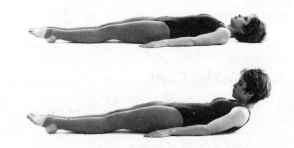

5

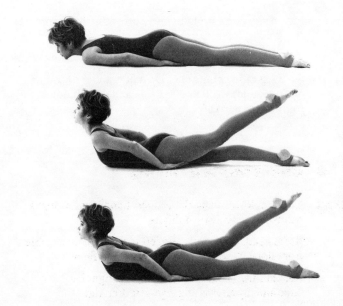

6

## 7  Side leg raising

**Start**  Lie on side, legs straight, lower arm stretched over head along floor, top arm used for balance.

Raise upper leg 18 to 24 inches. Lower to starting position.

**Count**  Each leg raise counts one. Do half number of counts raising left leg. Roll to other side and do half number of counts raising right leg.

CHART I

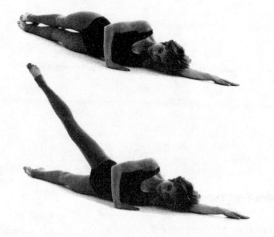

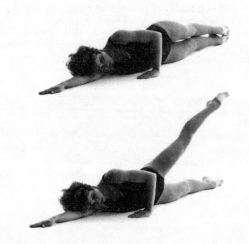

7

## 8  Push-ups

**Start**  Lie face down, legs straight and together, hands directly under shoulders.

Push body off floor in any way possible, keeping hands and knees in contact with floor. Sit back on heels. Lower body to floor.

**Count**  Each return to starting position counts one.

CHART I

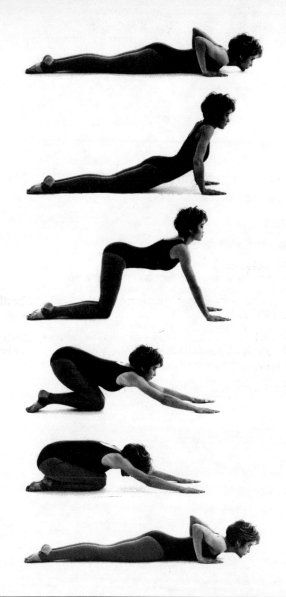

## 8

## 9  Leg lifting

**Start** Lie on back, legs straight and together, arms at sides, palms down.

Raise left leg until it is perpendicular to floor, or as close to this position as possible.

Lower and repeat with right leg.
Continue by alternating legs, left then right.

**Count**  Left plus right leg lifts count one.

CHART I

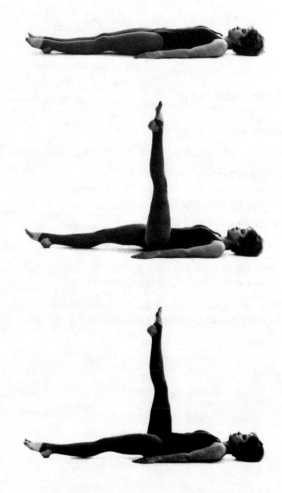

## 9

## 10  Run and hop

**Start**  Stand erect, feet together, arms at sides.

Starting with left leg, run in place raising feet at least four inches from floor.

(When running in place lift knees forward, do not merely kick heels backwards.)

**Count**  Each time left foot touches floor counts one.

After each fifty counts do ten hops.

**Hops**  Hopping is done so that both feet leave floor together. Try to hop at least four inches off floor each time.

*Note:* In all run-in-place exercises only running steps are counted towards completing exercise repetitions.

CHART I

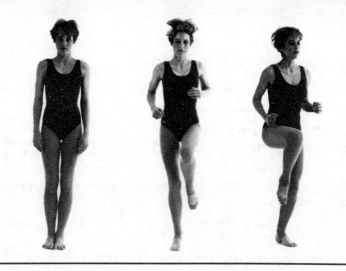

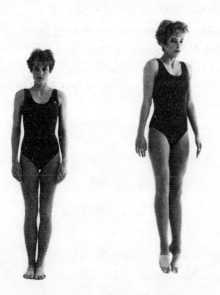

**10**

# Chart 2

*Handwritten column labels:* TOES · KNEES · SIDE BENDS · ARMS · ROCKING SIT-UPS · CHEST + LEG · SIDE LEG · KNEE PUSH-UPS · LEG-OVER · RUN+STRIDE JUMP

| Level | Exercise | | | | | | | | | | | |
|---|---|---|---|---|---|---|---|---|---|---|---|---|
| | 1 | 2 | 3 | 4 | 5 | 6 | 7 | 8 | 9 | 10 | 8a | 8b |
| 24 | 15 | 16 | 12 | 30 | 35 | 38 | 50 | 28 | 20 | 210 | 40 | 36 |
| 23 | 15 | 16 | 12 | 30 | 33 | 36 | 48 | 26 | 18 | 200 | 38 | 34 |
| 22 | 15 | 16 | 12 | 30 | 31 | 34 | 46 | 24 | 18 | 200 | 36 | 32 |
| 21 | 13 | 14 | 11 | 26 | 29 | 32 | 44 | 23 | 16 | 190 | 33 | 29 |
| 20 | 13 | 14 | 11 | 26 | 27 | 31 | 42 | 21 | 16 | 175 | 31 | 27 |
| 19 | 13 | 14 | 11 | 26 | 24 | 29 | 40 | 20 | 14 | 160 | 28 | 24 |
| 18 | 12 | 12 | 9 | 20 | 22 | 27 | 38 | 18 | 14 | 150 | 25 | 22 |
| 17 | 12 | 12 | 9 | 20 | 19 | 24 | 36 | 16 | 12 | 150 | 22 | 20 |
| 16 | 12 | 12 | 9 | 20 | 16 | 21 | 34 | 14 | 10 | 140 | 19 | 19 |
| 15 | 10 | 10 | 7 | 18 | 14 | 18 | 32 | 12 | 10 | 130 | 17 | 15 |
| 14 | 10 | 10 | 7 | 18 | 11 | 15 | 30 | 10 | 8 | 120 | 14 | 13 |
| 13 | 10 | 10 | 7 | 18 | 9 | 12 | 28 | 8 | 8 | 120 | 12 | 12 |
| Minutes for each exercise | | 2 | | | 2 | 1 | 1 | 2 | 1 | 3 | 1 | 1 |

Recommended number of days at each level ▢

## My Progress

| Level | Started | Finished | Comments |
|-------|---------|----------|----------|
| 24 | _____ | _____ | _____ |
| 23 | _____ | _____ | _____ |
| 22 | _____ | _____ | _____ |
| 22 | _____ | _____ | _____ |
| 21 | _____ | _____ | _____ |
| 20 | _____ | _____ | _____ |
| 19 | _____ | _____ | _____ |
| 18 | _____ | _____ | _____ |
| 17 | _____ | _____ | _____ |
| 16 | _____ | _____ | _____ |
| 15 | _____ | _____ | _____ |
| 14 | _____ | _____ | _____ |
| 13 | _____ | _____ | _____ |

|  | Date | Height | Weight | Waist | Hips | Bust |
|--|------|--------|--------|-------|------|------|
| My aim | _____ | _____ | _____ | _____ | _____ | _____ |
| Start | _____ | _____ | _____ | _____ | _____ | _____ |
| Finish | _____ | _____ | _____ | _____ | _____ | _____ |

## 1  Toe touching

**Start**    Stand erect, feet 12 inches apart, arms over head.

Bend forward to touch floor between feet.

Bob up and down touching floor a second time.

Return to starting position.

**Count**    Each return to starting position counts one.


## 2  Knee raising

**Start**    Stand erect, feet together, arms at sides.

Raise left knee as high as possible grasping knee and shin with hands. Pull leg against body. Keep back straight throughout. Lower foot to floor.

Repeat with right leg. Continue by alternating legs – left then right.

**Count**    Left and right knee raises count one.

CHART 2

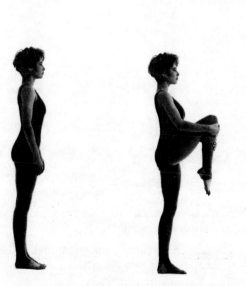

1

2

## 3  Lateral bending

**Start**  Stand erect, feet 12 inches apart, hands at sides.

Keeping back straight, bend sidewards from waist to left. Slide left hand down leg as far as possible. Bob up a few inches and press sidewards and down again.

Return to starting position and repeat same movements to right side. Continue by alternating to left then right.

**Count**  Bends to left and right count one.


## 4  Arm circling

**Start**  Stand erect, feet 12 inches apart, arms at sides.

Make large circles, with both arms at same time, backwards and round.

Do half the number of repetitions making backward circles and half making forward circles.

**Count**  Each full arm circle counts one.

CHART 2

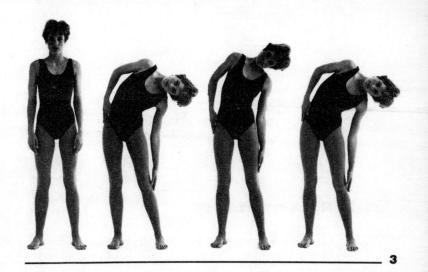

3

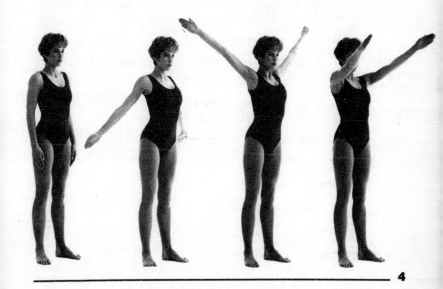

4

## 5  Rocking sit-ups

**Start**  Lie on back, knees bent, feet on floor, arms extended over head.

Swing arms forward and at same time thrust feet forward and move to sitting position. Reach forward, trying to touch toes with fingers.

Return to starting position.

**Count**  Each return to starting position counts one.

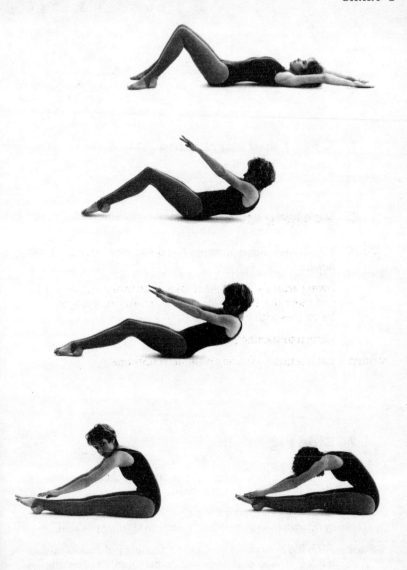

CHART 2

## 6 Chest and leg raising

**Start**  Lie face down, arms along sides, palms pressing against thighs

Raise head, shoulders, and legs as high as possible from floor. Keep legs straight.

Return to starting position.

**Count**  Each return to starting position counts one.


## 7 Side leg raising

**Start**  Lie on side, legs straight, lower arm stretched over head along floor, top arm used for balance.

Raise upper leg until it is perpendicular to floor or as close to this position as possible. Lower to starting position.

**Count**  Each leg rise counts one. Do half number of counts raising left leg. Roll to other side and do half number of counts raising right leg.

CHART 2

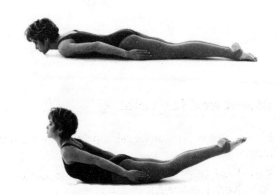

6

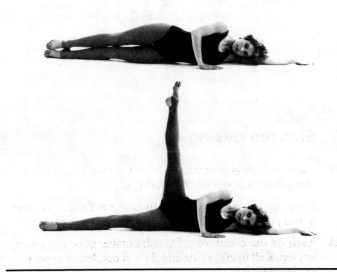

7

## 8  Knee push-ups

**Start**   Lie face down, legs straight and together, hands directly under shoulders.

Push body off floor until arms are straightened. Keep hands and knees in contact with floor. Try to keep body in straight line.

**Count**   Each return to starting position counts one.

CHART 2

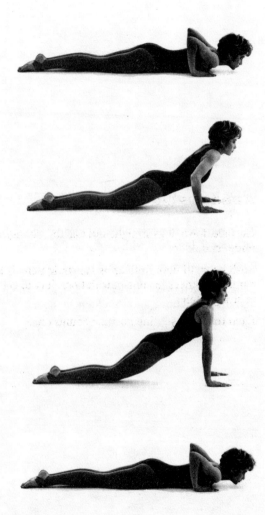

## 9 Leg-overs

**Start**  Lie on back, legs straight and together, arms stretched sidewards at shoulder level.

Raise right leg to perpendicular. Drop it across body, and try to touch left hand with toes.

Raise leg to perpendicular and return to starting position.

Repeat same movements with left leg. Keep body and legs straight throughout, and shoulders on floor.

**Count**  Each return to starting position counts one.

CHART 2

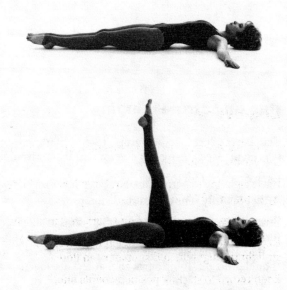

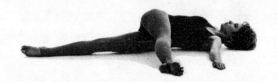

9

## 10 Run and stride jumping

**Start** Stand erect, feet together, arms at sides. Starting with left leg run in place raising feet at least four inches from floor.

**Count** Each time left foot touches floor counts one.

After each fifty runs do ten stride jumps.

**Stride** Stride jump starts with feet together, arms at sides.
**jump** Jump so that feet are about 18 inches apart when you land. At the same time as you jump, raise arms sidewards to shoulder height. Jump again so that feet are together and arms are at sides when you land.

CHART 2

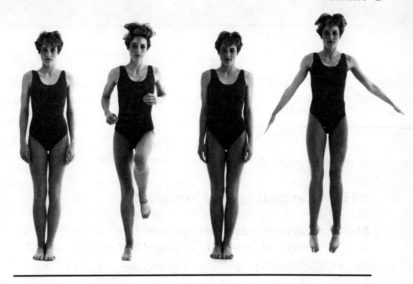

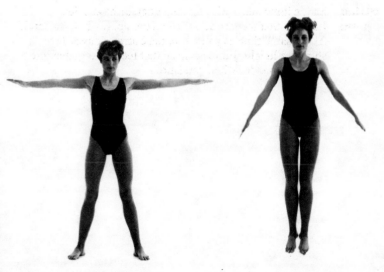

**10**

59

## Chart 3

| Level | 1 | 2 | 3 | 4 | 5 | 6 | 7 | 8 | 9 | 10 | 8a | 8b |
|---|---|---|---|---|---|---|---|---|---|---|---|---|
| | Exercise | | | | | | | | | | | |
| 36 | 15 | 22 | 18 | 40 | 42 | 40 | 60 | 40 | 20 | 240 | 32 | 38 |
| 35 | 15 | 22 | 18 | 40 | 41 | 39 | 60 | 39 | 20 | 230 | 30 | 36 |
| 34 | 15 | 22 | 18 | 40 | 40 | 38 | 58 | 37 | 19 | 220 | 29 | 34 |
| 33 | 13 | 20 | 16 | 36 | 39 | 36 | 58 | 35 | 19 | 210 | 27 | 33 |
| 32 | 13 | 20 | 16 | 36 | 37 | 36 | 56 | 34 | 18 | 200 | 25 | 31 |
| 31 | 13 | 20 | 16 | 36 | 35 | 34 | 56 | 32 | 16 | 200 | 24 | 30 |
| 30 | 12 | 18 | 14 | 30 | 33 | 33 | 54 | 30 | 15 | 190 | 23 | 28 |
| 29 | 12 | 18 | 14 | 30 | 32 | 31 | 54 | 29 | 14 | 180 | 21 | 26 |
| 28 | 12 | 18 | 14 | 30 | 31 | 30 | 52 | 27 | 12 | 170 | 20 | 25 |
| 27 | 10 | 16 | 12 | 24 | 29 | 30 | 52 | 25 | 11 | 160 | 19 | 23 |
| 26 | 10 | 16 | 12 | 24 | 27 | 29 | 50 | 23 | 9 | 150 | 17 | 21 |
| 25 | 10 | 16 | 12 | 24 | 26 | 28 | 48 | 22 | 8 | 140 | 16 | 20 |
| Minutes for each exercise | | 2 | | | 2 | 1 | 1 | 2 | 1 | 3 | 1 | 1 |

Recommended number of days at each level ☐

## My Progress

| Level | Started | Finished | Comments |
|-------|---------|----------|----------|
| 36 | _____ | _____ | _____ |
| 35 | _____ | _____ | _____ |
| 34 | _____ | _____ | _____ |
| 33 | _____ | _____ | _____ |
| 32 | _____ | _____ | _____ |
| 31 | _____ | _____ | _____ |
| 30 | _____ | _____ | _____ |
| 29 | _____ | _____ | _____ |
| 28 | _____ | _____ | _____ |
| 27 | _____ | _____ | _____ |
| 26 | _____ | _____ | _____ |
| 25 | _____ | _____ | _____ |

|  | Date | Height | Weight | Waist | Hips | Bust |
|--|------|--------|--------|-------|------|------|
| My aim | _____ | _____ | _____ | _____ | _____ | _____ |
| Start | _____ | _____ | _____ | _____ | _____ | _____ |
| Finish | _____ | _____ | _____ | _____ | _____ | _____ |

## 1  Toe touching

**Start**  Stand erect, feet about 16 inches apart, arms over head.

Bend down to touch floor outside left foot. Bob up and down to touch floor between feet. Bob again and bend to touch floor outside right foot.

Return to starting position.

**Count**  Each return to starting position counts one.

CHART 3

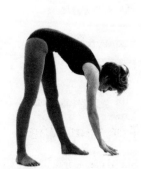

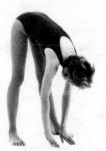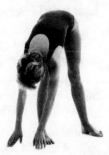

1

## 2  Knee raising

**Start**    Stand erect, feet together, arms at sides.

Raise left knee as high as possible, grasping knee and shin with hands.

Pull leg against body. Keep back straight throughout. Lower foot to floor.

Repeat with right leg. Continue by alternating legs – left then right.

**Count**    Left and right knee raises count one.

## 3  Lateral bending

**Start**    Stand erect, feet 12 inches apart, right arm extended over head, bent at elbow.

Keeping back straight, bend sidewards from waist to left. Slide left hand down leg as far as possible, at the same time press to left with right arm.

Return to starting position and change arm positions. Repeat to right. Continue by alternating to left then right.

**Count**    Bends to left and right count one.

CHART 3

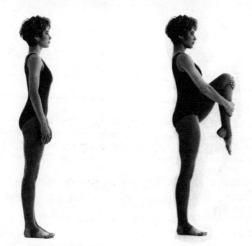

**2**

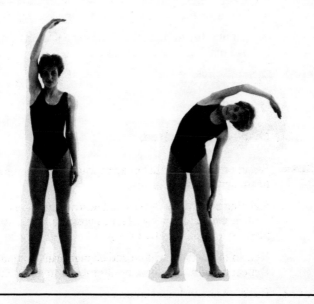

**3**

## 4 Arm circling

**Start**  Stand erect, feet 12 inches apart, arms at sides.

Make large circles with arms in a windmill action – one arm following the other and both moving at same time.

Do half number of repetitions making backward circles and half making forward circles.

**Count**  Each full circle by both arms counts one.

CHART 3

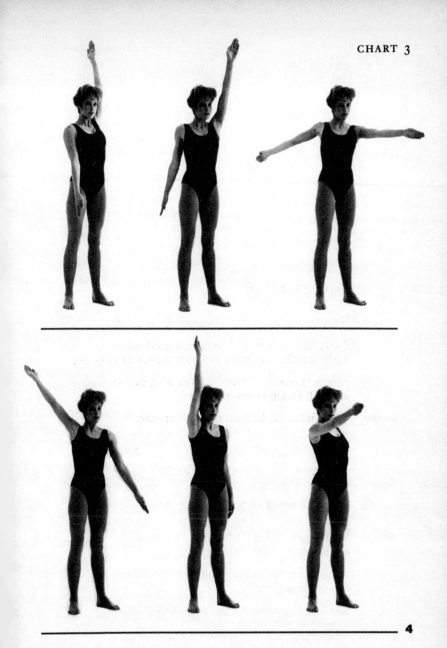

**4**

## 5  Sit-ups

**Start**  Lie on back, legs straight and together, arms along sides.

Keeping back as straight as possible, move to a sitting position.

Slide hands along legs during this movement finally reaching forward to try to touch toes with fingers.

Return to starting position.

**Count**  Each return to starting position counts one.


## 6  Chest and leg raising

**Start**  Lie face down, legs straight and together, arms stretched sidewards at shoulder level.

Raise entire upper body and both legs from floor as high as possible.

Keep legs straight. Return to starting position.

**Count**  Each return to starting position counts one.

CHART 3

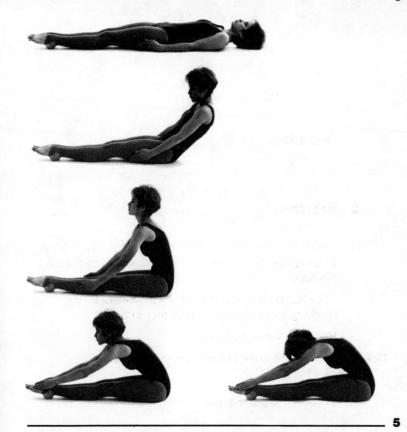

**5**

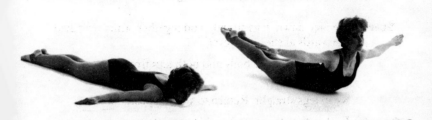

**6**

69

## 7 Side leg raising

**Start**  Lie on side, legs straight, lower arm stretched over head along floor, top arm used for balance.

Raise upper leg until it is perpendicular to floor. Lower to starting position.

**Count**  Each leg raise counts one. Do half number of counts raising left leg. Roll to other side and do half number of counts raising right leg.

## 8 Elbow push-ups

**Start**  Lie face down, legs straight and together, elbows directly under shoulders, forearms along floor, and hands clasped together.

Raise body from floor by straightening it from head to heels.

In the up position, body is in a straight line and elbows, forearms, and toes are in contact with floor.

Lower to starting position. Keep head up throughout.

**Count**  Each return to starting position counts one.

CHART 3

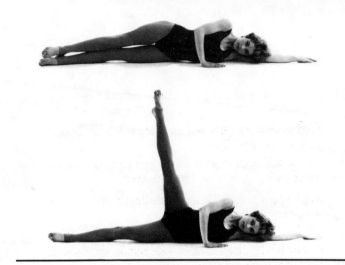

7

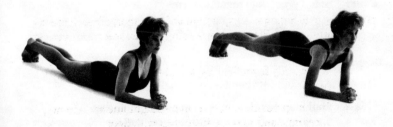

8

## 9 Leg-overs — Tuck

**Start** Lie on back, legs straight and together, arms stretched sidewards at shoulder level, palms down.

Raise both legs from floor, bending at hips and knees until in a tuck position.

Lower legs to left, keeping knees together and both shoulders on floor.

Raise legs and lower to floor on right side.

Raise until perpendicular to floor and return to starting position. Keep knees close to abdomen throughout.

**Count** Each return to starting position counts one.

## 10 Run and half knee bends

**Start** Stand erect, feet together, arms at sides.

Starting with left leg, run in place raising feet at least six inches from floor.

**Count** Each time left foot touches floor counts one.

After each fifty counts do ten half knee bends.

**Half knee bends** Half knee bends start with hands on hips, feet together, body erect. Bend at knees and hips, lowering body until thigh and calf form an angle of about 110 degrees. Do not bend knees past a right angle. Keep back straight. Return to starting position.

CHART 3

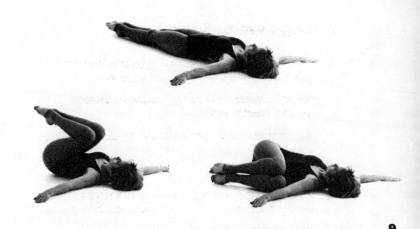

9

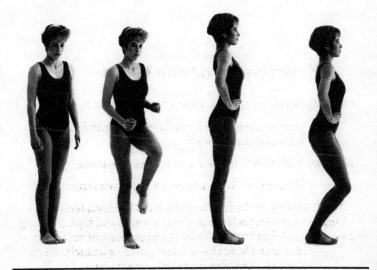

10

# Chart 4

| Level | Exercise | | | | | | | | | |
|---|---|---|---|---|---|---|---|---|---|---|
| | **1** | **2** | **3** | **4** | **5** | **6** | **7** | **8** | **9** | **10** |
| **48** | 15 | 26 | 15 | 32 | 48 | 46 | 58 | 30 | 16 | 230 |
| **47** | 15 | 26 | 15 | 32 | 45 | 45 | 56 | 27 | 15 | 220 |
| **46** | 15 | 26 | 15 | 32 | 44 | 44 | 54 | 24 | 14 | 210 |
| **45** | 13 | 24 | 14 | 30 | 42 | 43 | 52 | 21 | 13 | 200 |
| **44** | 13 | 24 | 14 | 30 | 40 | 42 | 50 | 19 | 13 | 190 |
| **43** | 13 | 24 | 14 | 30 | 38 | 40 | 48 | 16 | 12 | 175 |
| **42** | 12 | 22 | 12 | 28 | 35 | 39 | 46 | 13 | 10 | 160 |
| **41** | 12 | 22 | 12 | 28 | 32 | 38 | 44 | 11 | 9 | 150 |
| **40** | 12 | 22 | 12 | 28 | 30 | 38 | 40 | 9 | 8 | 140 |
| **39** | 10 | 20 | 10 | 26 | 29 | 36 | 38 | 8 | 7 | 130 |
| **38** | 10 | 20 | 10 | 26 | 27 | 35 | 36 | 7 | 6 | 115 |
| **37** | 10 | 20 | 10 | 26 | 25 | 34 | 34 | 6 | 5 | 100 |
| Minutes for each exercise | | 2 | | | 2 | 1 | 1 | 2 | 1 | 3 |

Recommended number of days at each level ☐

74

## My Progress

| Level | Started | Finished | Comments |
|-------|---------|----------|----------|
| 48 | _____ | _____ | _____ |
| 47 | _____ | _____ | _____ |
| 46 | _____ | _____ | _____ |
| 46 | _____ | _____ | _____ |
| 45 | _____ | _____ | _____ |
| 44 | _____ | _____ | _____ |
| 43 | _____ | _____ | _____ |
| 42 | _____ | _____ | _____ |
| 41 | _____ | _____ | _____ |
| 40 | _____ | _____ | _____ |
| 39 | _____ | _____ | _____ |
| 38 | _____ | _____ | _____ |
| 37 | _____ | _____ | _____ |

|  | Date | Height | Weight | Waist | Hips | Bust |
|--------|------|--------|--------|-------|------|------|
| My aim | _____ | _____ | _____ | _____ | _____ | _____ |
| Start | _____ | _____ | _____ | _____ | _____ | _____ |
| Finish | _____ | _____ | _____ | _____ | _____ | _____ |

# 1  Toe touching

**Start** Stand erect, feet about 16 inches apart, arms over head.

Bend down to touch floor outside left foot. Bob up and down to touch floor between feet. Bob again touching floor between feet once more. Bob and bend to touch floor outside right foot.

Return to starting position.

**Count** Each return to starting position counts one.

CHART 4

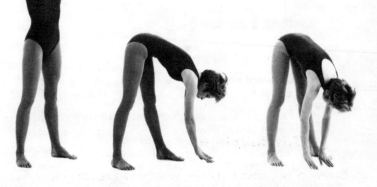

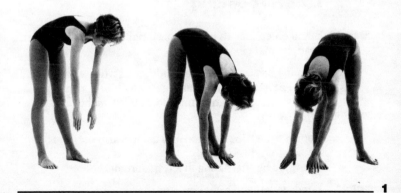

1

## 2  Knee raising

**Start**  Stand erect, feet together, arms at sides.

Raise left knee as high as possible, grasping knee and shin with hands.

Pull leg against body. Keep back straight throughout. Lower foot to floor.

Repeat with right leg. Continue by alternating legs – left then right.

**Count**  Left and right knee raises count one.


## 3  Lateral bending

**Start**  Stand erect, feet 12 inches apart, right arm extended over head, bent at elbow.

Keeping back straight, bend sidewards from waist to left. Slide left hand down leg as far as possible, at same time press to left with right arm. Bob up a few inches and press to left again.

Return to starting position and change arm positions. Repeat to right.
Continue by alternating to left then right.

**Count**  Bends to left and right count one.

CHART 4

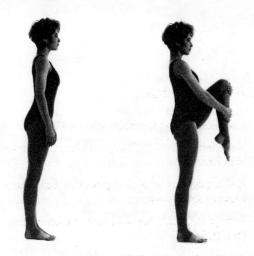

2

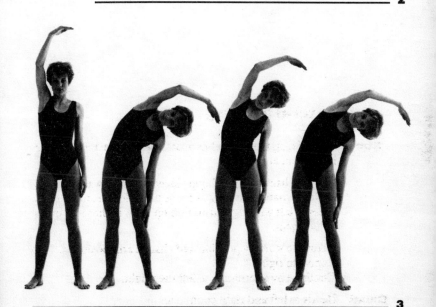

3

## 4  Arm flinging

**Start**  Stand erect, feet 12 inches apart, upper arms extended sidewards at shoulder level, elbows bent, outstretched fingers touching in front of chest.

Press elbows backward and upward. Do not let elbows drop.

Return arms to starting position and then fling hands and arms outward, backward, and upward as far as possible.

Return to starting position.

**Count**  Count one after each arm fling.

## 5  Sit-ups

**Start**  Lie on back, legs straight and together, hands behind head.

Move to sitting position. Keep feet on floor (support may be used if necessary) and back straight.

Lower body to starting position.

**Count**  Each return to starting position counts one.

CHART 4

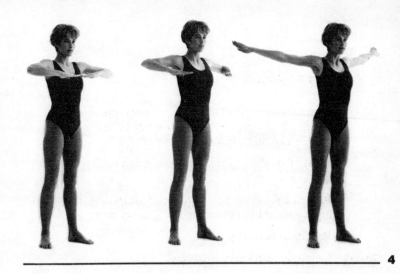

4

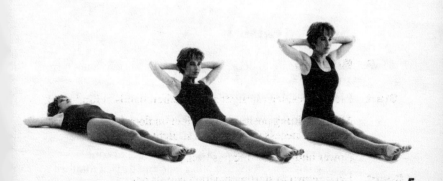

5

## 6  Chest and leg raising

**Start**  Lie face down, legs straight and together, hands behind head.

Raise entire upper body and both legs from floor as high as possible. Keep legs straight.

Return to starting position.

**Count**  Each return to starting position counts one.

## 7  Side leg raising

**Start**  With right side to floor, support weight on right hand (arm straight) and side of right foot, using left hand for assistance in balance if necessary.

Raise left leg until it is parallel with floor. Lower leg to starting position.

**Count**  Each leg raise counts one. Do half number of counts raising left leg. Change to other side and do half number of counts raising right leg.

CHART 4

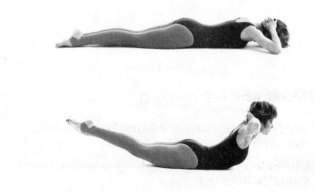

6

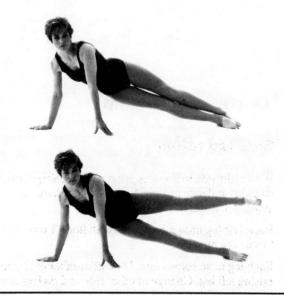

7

## 8  Push-ups

**Start**   Lie face down, legs straight and together, toes turned under, hands directly under shoulders.

Push up from hands and toes until arms are fully extended.

Keep body and legs in a straight line. Return to touch chest to floor and repeat.

**Count**   Each time chest touches floor count one.


## 9  Leg-overs — Straight

**Start**   Lie on back, legs straight and together, arms stretched sidewards at shoulder level, palms down.

Raise both legs until they are perpendicular to floor, keeping them straight and together.

Lower legs to left, trying to touch left hand with toes.

Raise to perpendicular and lower to right side.

Raise again to perpendicular and return to starting position.

**Count**   Each return to starting position counts one.

CHART 4

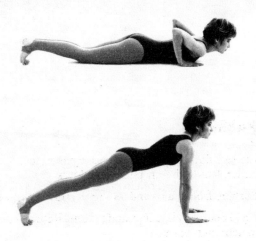

8

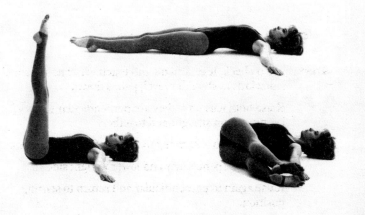

9

## 10  Run and semi-squat jumps

**Start**   Stand erect, feet together, arms at sides.

Starting with left leg, run in place raising feet at least six inches from floor.

**Count**   Each time left foot touches floor counts one.

After each fifty counts do ten semi-squat jumps.

**Semi-squat jumps**   Drop to a half crouch position with hands on knees and arms straight. Keep back as straight as possible, one foot slightly ahead of the other. Jump to upright position with body straight and feet leaving floor. Reverse position of feet before landing, return to half crouch, and repeat.

CHART 4

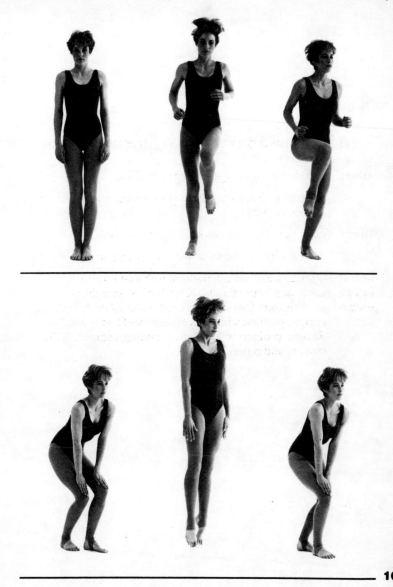

10

# Supplementary Exercises

On the following pages the supplementary exercises for feet, ankles, and posture are illustrated and described. If you wish to do these exercises they are to be included in your regular programme between Exercises Eight and Nine and are numbered Eight A and Eight B.

## 8a  Feet and ankles

**Start**  Sit on floor, legs straight and about six inches apart, hands behind body for support, feet relaxed.

Press toes away from body as far as possible.

Bring toes towards body hooking feet as much as possible.

Relax feet.

**Count**  Each return to relaxed state counts one.


## 8b  Posture

**Start**  Sit on floor, knees bent, feet on floor, hands clasped about knees, head bent forward, and body relaxed.

Straighten body and lift head to look directly ahead. Pull in muscles of abdomen.

Relax to starting position.

**Count**  Each return to starting position counts one.

CHART I

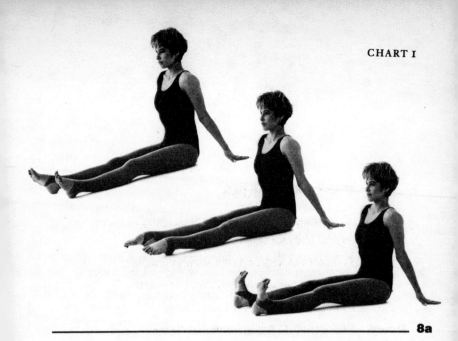

8a

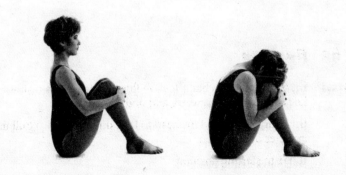

8b

## 8a  Feet and ankles

**Start**  Sit on floor, legs straight and heels about 14 inches apart, hands behind body for support, feet relaxed.

Move feet so that toes make large circular movements. Press out and around and in and towards the body.

Do half number of counts moving toes in one direction, then reverse for remainder of counts.

**Count**  Each time toes describe a full circle counts one.

## 8b  Posture

**Start**  Lie on back, knees bent, feet on floor, arms slightly to side. Relax muscles of trunk.

Press lower part of back to floor by tightening muscles of abdomen and back.

Relax to starting position.

**Count**  Each return to starting position counts one.

CHART 2

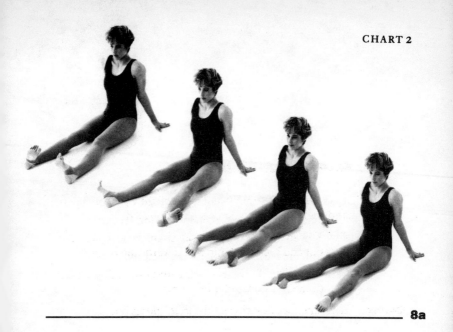

8a

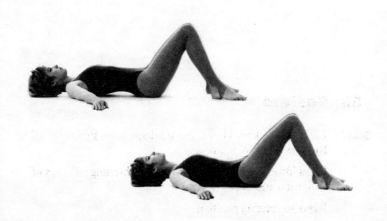

8b

## 8a  Feet and ankles

**Start**  Stand erect, arms at sides, feet about 12 inches apart.

First raise up on to toes, then lower until feet are flat on floor.

Next roll outward on sides of feet, then roll feet so that outside edge of foot is off floor.

Return to starting position.

**Count**  Each return to starting position counts one.


## 8b  Posture

**Start**  Lie on back, legs straight and together, arms slightly to side. Relax muscles of trunk.

Press lower part of back to floor by tightening muscles of abdomen and back.

Relax to starting position.

**Count**  Each return to starting position counts one.

CHART 3

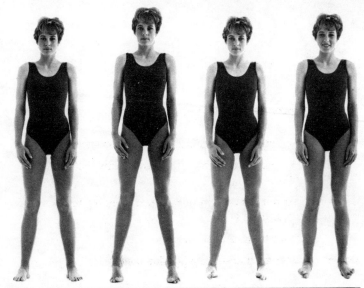

8a

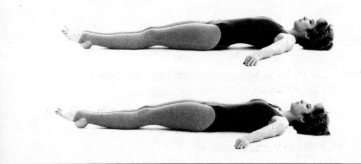

8b